SURVIVAL GUIDE FOR DEMENTIA CAREGIVERS.

NANCY JUDY

COPYRIGHT

Copyright © 2021 by NANCY JUDY: All rights reserved. This book or any portion thereof may not be reproduced or used in any manner whatsoever without the express written permission of the author except for the use of brief quotations in a book review.

TABLE OF CONTENTS

INTRODUCTION **3**

CHAPTER 1 .... **5**
   LET'S START FROM THE BEGINNING 5

CHAPTER 2 .... **12**
   CAREGIVER'S JOB DESCRIPTION 12

CHAPTER 3 .... **17**
   TYPES OF DEMENTIA. 17

CHAPTER 4 .... **32**
   THE NASTY SIDE OF DEMENTIA. 32

CHAPTER 5 .... **35**
   SYMPTOMS OF CAREGIVER BURNOUT 35

CHAPTER 6 .... **40**
   ACTIVITIES TO EASE DEMENTIA. 40

CHAPTER 7 .... **45**
   CARING FOR DEMENTIA PATIENTS 45

CHAPTER 8 .... **48**
   THERAPY FOR DEMENTIA CAREGIVERS 48

CONCLUSION **53**

INTRODUCTION

Dementia is a common condition experienced by most ageing people. There are nearly 45 million persons living with dementia worldwide and this figure is predicted to multiply every twenty years. Alzheimer's disease is the most well-known kind of dementia. It starts with a gentle cognitive decline which gradually leads to memory loss and the inability to recognize the environment. This emphasizes why it is important to understand what it is and how we can manage its symptoms effectively.

Dementia controls the mind, thought, memory, and language. It can truly influence an individual's capacity to complete day by day activities. It is alarming to know that in 2020, about 5.8 million Americans were living with Alzheimer's disease. These statistics do not just cover the elderly population, the younger population are at risk also. The elderly population tend to experience dementia from the age of 65 years. This number is projected to almost significantly increase to 14 million individuals by 2060. Manifestations of the illness would first be able to show up after age 60, and this gets worse with age.

Changes in brain activity can start a very long time before the manifestations of dementia show up. Memory issues are regularly one of the principal noticeable indications of Alzheimer's sickness and related dementias. Age is the most popular danger factor for dementia. Researchers don't yet completely comprehend what causes dementia, but there are likely factors that contribute to this sickness which we would be examining in this book.

Most times people living with dementia or with Alzheimer's sickness have their primary caregivers as relatives. The vast majority of caregivers readily give care to their friends, family and companions, with Alzheimer's sickness. Home care can be a troublesome assignment and may get overpowering now and again. Every day brings new difficulties as the illness deteriorates, individuals living with Alzheimer's sickness regularly need more escalated care. Providing care can have positive perspectives such as creating bonding time with a loved one, but the complication that could come from caring with a relative with dementia is not an easy battle for any caregiver that has very little knowledge about the disease. Caring for people with dementia is never an easy task to deal with, which is why this book gives a practical guide on the best ways to help caregivers become knowledgeable to give the best care to persons living with dementia.

CHAPTER 1
LET'S START FROM THE BEGINNING

The word 'dementia' is derived from the Latin word *demens* which simply means 'out of one's mind. Dementia is almost as old as mankind. In the late 18th century, with advancement in neurology, brain scans were carried out and this was when it was discovered that the disease could cause a degeneration in the brain cells. Dementia in itself is not a disease but a clinical syndrome which refers to a group of symptom that works together in a similar pattern. Dementia is a class of symptoms that causes a deterioration in two brain activities e.g. thinking and judgement. This is why Dementia can take many forms that will shortly be discussed. Dementia is simply a generic term for a brain disease or condition that causes a deterioration in one's ability to think, comprehend, learn, calculate and remember vital information. There are various types of dementia. The symptoms could either be very pronounced or progressive in nature. Dementia is also linked with sudden emotional changes, temperaments or changes in behaviour. Dementia is caused by Alzheimer's disease and cerebrovascular disease.

Alzheimer's disease is more often than not, responsible for the development of dementia in older people. It is a degenerative disease of the brain nerves over time or shrinking of the brain nerves distorting memory and other mental functions such as thinking and giving good judgments. Alzheimer's disease (AD) gets worse over time as no specific cure has been found for it. However, its symptoms are treatable. It is caused by the development of plaques and tangles in the hippocampus and cerebral cortex deep in the brain-The hippocampus is the region where memories are inscribed while the cerebral cortex helps with thoughts and making decisions. AD usually occurs or in the early '60s of a person life. However, recent research has confirmed its occurrence in younger individuals in their late 30's or early 40's. Alzheimer's disease was founded and named after the scientist who discovered it; Alois Alzheimer.

Plaques in the brain are not the regular plaques we know that form on the teeth. In this case, plaques in the brain are caused by the formation of protein fragments called beta-amyloid in areas between the nerve cells of the brain. Tangles in the brain are caused by another protein called tau which has twisted fibres that develop in the brain over time. It is after the nerves cells are destroyed or shrunk that memory loss and other symptoms begin to occur. People with AD find it very difficult to perform regular day to day tasks that they used to do before, such as taking a bath, cooking driving, buying groceries and many more. They can also get very aggressive at times. This is why caregivers are needed.

Alzheimer's disease is not normal in ageing people as most believed by most people. Not every ageing person develops it. With the estimated discovery of over 200,000 Americans living with AD (65 or older); there are still some individual going through the normal ageing process. Signs and symptoms of ageing and Alzheimer's disease are quite similar. Research has shown that 90% of elderly people develop plaques and tangles as well. The only difference is people living with AD, develop far more plaques and tangles in a similar pattern that can be identified starting from the hippocampus and spreading out to other areas in the brain

Ageing people may lose things sometimes and find them later. People with AD lose things more often and may never be able to find them again as their ability to recollect has been distorted. This also explains why they also find it difficult to recall new information. You tell them something new, and they do not remember the next minute.

People living with AD find it difficult to have a conversational flow so it's hard to communicate with them. Ageing people, on the other hand, may forget words to use. AD causes general confusion and disorganization in a person's life. They forget where they keep things, forget to pay their monthly bills and even forget the time of the year. Ageing people on the other hand may occasionally misplace things, skip a monthly bill and forget today's date. However, they can still perform basic day to day tasks like cooking, bathing, eating and other things that may a major problem for people living with AD.

Signs of Dementia: The first thing any caregiver must understand are the signs of this disease. Dementia can be identified by many related signs such as forgetting the names of close friends and family, occasional aggression, impaired judgement, difficulty in communicating, restlessness, mood swings, and other strange behavioural and social changes that are somewhat usual. I once visited a hospital and overheard a patient call his caregiver his child, then I wasn't so knowledgeable about dementia but I knew that patient was having a bit of memory loss. There was no need for me to assume that patient had dementia because I have not seen the clinical diagnosis to ascertain the patient suffering from dementia, this is one of the major thing caregivers need to know, the signs has to be visible not just your thoughts. The early signs of dementia range from the following impairments: difficulties in communication, reasoning, speaking, focus and memory loss. Don't just assume your loved one has dementia because they have a little symptom, please consult a trained physician before making an assumption, as human life is very precious to bank on mere assumptions.

A person suffering from dementia could experience short term memory changes, this is a reverse condition where the person could remember events from a week or month ago but not the present day of what they had for breakfast. I have a friend who takes care of himself he is in his late 80's the day I had a video call with him I saw a lot of tags, what we term vision boards reminding him to do several activities, although he never sounds like someone that has dementia, this is one of the tricky part caregivers need to note. Subtle short term memory loss could be managed through vision boards or sometimes it could just be the brain cleaning up some space. When you need to act as a home giver is when current activities cannot be remembered by the person suffering from dementia. Sometimes a person with dementia could forget where they kept their keys, their activities for the day, appointments, faces of loved ones, hobbies but remembers what happened years ago. Caregivers need to be very patient handling people with dementia as most times aggression arises from memory loss, the patient could see their caregiver as a stranger and thereby tend towards demeaning or violent behaviours, please stay calm and think of the best way to bring pea e into the storm.

It is difficult for someone with dementia to have difficulties finding the right words whenever they are engaged in conversations, I have heard of a granny call her newborn granddaughter ugly and fat, it is just a hard time for her to find the right words to express herself. Sometimes caregivers find it a bit difficult to understand what their patient is trying to say because they cannot properly explain with the right words that is why you need to be patient, kind, understanding, and smart as a trained caregiver.

Mood swings are a common phenomenon in a person suffering from dementia. In the early stages of dementia, depression tends to set in along with mood changes, it is the duty of a caregiver to identify the quick varying changes in mood from over-excited to depressed mood, shy to outgoing mood, happiness to angry mood and the immediate change in personality traits. Dementia affects a person's judgment that is why it is very common to observe fast mood changes. I watched a rending video where a caregiver had a video proof to show his client was violent towards him, in that video the patient had no empathy for his violent behaviour. My major inputs from that video were first, the fact that the caregiver breached the Non-disclosure agreement with their patient and secondly the fact that the caregiver failed to realise the patient has no empathy as people suffering from dementia are often emotionally flat and show several episodes of mood changes. The goal of this book is to prepare caregivers to always be alert and find a balance between burnout and working on the job.

As a trusted caregiver one early sign to note in your patient is the difficulty they may experience carrying out easy tasks that is not the time to increase their burden but to help them scale through such tasks. Get ready or prepare your mind to find a solution when your patient cannot follow your daily routines, they could either be confused or experiencing some difficulties. Confusion happens due to memory lapses, you could observe that find it difficult to follow the storyline of their favourite TV programs. As a caregiver always show empathy to your patients failing sense of direction, being repetitive or struggling to adapt to change, just help them overcome the hurdles.

This chapter has explained in details the most significant early symptoms to note in people before terming them to have dementia. However, it is worthy to note that dementia varies in people, especially as they get older. It is important to care for a patient, friend, or family who has been clinically diagnosed with dementia with adequate resources and knowledge. Every caregiver needs to undergo professional training or certification to help improve the lives of those at risk or suffering from dementia.

CHAPTER 2
CAREGIVER'S JOB DESCRIPTION

When interacting with a patient who has Alzheimer's disease, caregiver tasks can vary. This disease brings with it a new set of tasks for caregivers, which may be both tough and gratifying. You must be clear about your circumstances and responsibilities as a caretaker. You'll need specific care information if you live with someone who has dementia and have to help them with day-to-day duties. Caregivers also have different perspectives on how their caregiving affects their sense of self and feelings like guilt, blame, responsibility, and accountability. Caregivers can be teenagers, young adults, middle-aged people, or even the elderly. They could be any gender female or male. They could be caring for a person of the same or opposite gender. They could be wealthy, middle-class, or a regular person. They could be well-educated and employed, or illiterate and unemployed. Expectations of them, as well as the resources accessible to them, vary. This has an impact on how people receive care and what they can do about it. You'll need to think about how you'll provide care now and in the future as dementia progresses. You must be prepared to provide care for a long period. If you try to do too many things at first, you will become physically and emotionally exhausted and unable to care for the individual as they become more reliant on you.

Caregiving entails providing physical assistance for a variety of tasks. It entails dealing with emotionally distressed dementia patients. Learn how to communicate with those who have dementia. Learn how to assist children with daily tasks while encouraging them to be as self-sufficient as possible. Frequently, they may cause harm to themselves or others. They may become enraged, wander, or ignore themselves. Learn how to remain cool in the face of adversity. At different stages of dementia, different care skills are required. When people with dementia become bedridden, for example, you'll require home nursing skills like how to change a dirty sheet and how to avoid pressure sores. Dementia care necessitates a wide range of caring abilities. Caring is often challenging since you must assist someone who may not comprehend or comply with you. Support groups and specialists can assist you in determining which topics are most beneficial to you. They may be able to assist you in obtaining important information. Reading books and watching training videos are both options.

The primary role of an Alzheimer's caregiver is to raise knowledge and comprehension of the condition, as well as how it affects the patient they're caring for. Alzheimer's is a disease that progresses through many stages and presentations. Memory loss, full loss of motor skills, unpredictable conduct, and difficulty to communicate are all possible symptoms. The caregiver can build a care strategy and set priorities by understanding the disease, the stage the patient is in, and how the patient is affected. Other elements to consider include housing environment, family relationships, and financial well-being.

Basic Aid: At its most basic level, caring for an Alzheimer's patient is providing basic support and assistance with daily activities. Depending on the patient and how far the condition has progressed, different levels of assistance may be required. Bathing, grooming, dressing, and eating assistance are all frequent chores. Caregivers frequently provide transportation and walking assistance. In general, the caregiver must ensure the patient's physical safety, especially since Alzheimer's disease can induce erratic behaviour, wandering, and poor motor skills and coordination.

Maintain Their Safety: Among the various responsibilities of a caregiver, guaranteeing the client's safety is one of the most important. Because some Alzheimer's patients have a proclivity for wandering away from home, caregivers should keep a close eye on their patients. Ensure that all doors are locked and that the client's neighbours are aware of his or her habits. Other tasks of the caregiver include ensuring the safety of the home; consider installing childproof locks on cupboards and doors, closely monitoring the use of cookware and the stove, keeping medicine locked up, and so on.

Stick to a Schedule: Establishing a schedule by performing your caregiving chores (eating, bathing, watching specific TV shows, etc.) at the same time each day can assist. Even taking the client to the bathroom at the same time each day can help establish regularity and reduce the risk of mishaps.

Be Calm and Patient: When working with Alzheimer's patients, it's critical to have a cool, calm, and collected demeanour when completing routine caregiver tasks. Seniors with Alzheimer's disease occasionally suffer "off days" when they are disconnected from the present. To avoid further irritating the client, it's critical to be patient and understanding during these moments.

Personal management: Caregivers assist individuals with Alzheimer's disease in managing their lives in a broader sense. One frequent responsibility is to establish a schedule and a routine. In one way or another, most Alzheimer's sufferers are still part of a larger community. They may have financial commitments, correspondence to attend to, activities to attend, and medical appointments to keep track of. Alzheimer's patients' caregivers aid them in meeting these commitments by assisting with organization and logistics. Caregivers may also assist an Alzheimer's patient in achieving personal goals such as writing memoirs, attending family gatherings, or reconnecting with old friends.

Emotional Support: For people with Alzheimer's disease, the disease is frightening, unpleasant, and unsettling. Emotional assistance and genuine social involvement are two of an Alzheimer's patient's most pressing demands. These things can be provided by the caregiver, who has a good emotional impact on the patient's life. Patients with Alzheimer's confront numerous obstacles to regular social participation, and isolation and melancholy can hasten the disease's progression. One of the most valuable services that a caregiver can provide is emotional support and commitment to serve.

CHAPTER 3
TYPES OF DEMENTIA.

Brain activity changes as we grow older. Those close to us such as our family, friends and loved ones are quick to see changes in memory, conduct, or capacities before they become full-blown. Some people experience cognitive decline as they mature or advance in age, not all brain decline is a cause for worry, but when the noticeable signs are very pronounced please consult a trained physician to discover the reason. Early intervention allows looking for treatment and plan for what's to come.

Dementia is the side effects of memory loss that influences the capacity to think, mingle, and remember. It causes disarray and a serious lack of critical thinking and language abilities. For the most part, individuals with dementia have serious struggles that affect their daily life.

Dementia influences individuals over age 65. Individuals with a direct relation who had dementia are bound to get it than those with no family background. When you notice a friend or family member has dementia, please ensure they visit a specialist who works in treating patients with dementia. Dementia can be a difficult encounter for everybody concerned. At the point when a friend or family member starts to give indications of decreasing psychological capacities, relatives may not comprehend the complexity of dealing with the sickness. Dementia can't be characterized by one sign or indication. The person in question may turn out to be more enthusiastic than expected or show indications of sorrow or outrage. Dementia advances in stages. It is imperative to understand the different stages and always seek medical advice as a caregiver.

Some experts do not refer to dementia as sickness or illness they tend to refer to it as a cognitive disability or memory loss. Neurologist term dementia as a cognitive disability, this means that caring for people with dementia should not be a scary adventure, it should be more of managing or helping someone with dementia cope and enjoy their life. States of mind are erratic when managing dementia. An individual can be restless and crying one second and fly into an irate fury the following. There are sure triggers that may cause these disturbing scenes. Dementia is like one's psyche playing several pranks on him, or her. There is a need to help people struggling with this illness adapt to changes. This chapter would focus on the types of dementia to help caregivers know the most suitable form of care to help manage this disability.

Alzheimer's disease: This is the most common type of dementia. Nearly 80% of people living with dementia have Alzheimer's disease. This disease is progressive in nature and is usually characterized by loss of memory and difficulty in communication. These symptoms worsen over time. Dementia is cognitive deficiencies in personality, judgement, memory loss, communication difficulties and the major cause is Alzheimer's disease. Most scientist term Alzheimer's disease as a type of early dementia symptom. Alzheimer's disease is very mild at the beginning, then it progresses to control the brain's ability to think, memorize, and communicate. The most common type of dementia is Alzheimer's disease it increases with age. The early signs of Alzheimer's disease may be invisible to everyone except the person suffering from the disease and those closest to them, the symptoms may be misdiagnosed as normal ageing changes. Alzheimer's disease is a brain disorder that causes memory loss, confusion, personality changes, and the gradual loss of independence. In some people, this disease progresses quickly, while in others, it progresses slowly. People with this disease experience memory loss and confusion these symptoms could start mild and worsen over time. Changes in the brain begin years before a person exhibits symptoms of this disease. This stage is known as preclinical Alzheimer disease, and it can last for years. Mild forgetfulness is one of the symptoms at this stage. This may appear to be the mild forgetfulness that comes with ageing. However, it may also include difficulties with concentration such as: recalling a name, managing and organizing. Genes, environment, lifestyle, and overall health all have a role to play in Alzheimer's disease. Treatment is frequently focused on slowing the process and ensuring a good quality of life. Caregivers can help reduce the progression of this sickness by ensuring the patient is always in a good and safe environment.

To begin care for someone with Alzheimer's disease the early signs and symptoms has to be carefully monitored, one of the vital things to look out for is Memory loss, poor decision-making abilities that interfere with daily life. In the early stages of this disease forgetting daily routines is one of the things caregivers have to help their patients remember. Planning or problem-solving difficulties could be experienced by those suffering from this disease. People suffering from Alzheimer's disease frequently struggle to complete daily tasks. They may have difficulty driving to a familiar location, pay less attention to grooming, difficulty following or joining a conversation, lose track of dates, place objects in unusual places, find it difficult organizing a grocery list, difficulties with balance or reading, mood swings and personality changes, struggle to follow a familiar recipe or keep track of monthly bills. They may have difficulty concentrating and may take much longer to complete tasks they did flawlessly.

Caregivers must always be aware of memory lapses in patients with Alzheimer's disease, as the disease progresses there are

Increasing difficulties for the patients in learning new things or keeping up with routines, they sometimes may forget their names or family members. It is important to caregivers know what to expect in patients with advanced Alzheimer's disease personality changes such as delusions, paranoia, or hallucinations, could come as the downside of dementia. Not all caregivers have the physical strength to tackle advanced personality changes like hallucinations, this is the time to consult a trained specialist to know the next step of immediate action to take. Always keeping tabs on a patient or taking notes would help determine the cause of the delusions. As a caregiver please always know the real condition of your patient to determine if you are mentally, physically or emotionally ready to tackle any challenges that might arise. To make a diagnosis, healthcare providers usually conduct memory tests to determine how well the person's brain functions. Brain scans, such as MRI, CT, or PET scans, may be included in these tests. Treatment options vary depending on a person's medical history, age, symptoms, overall health, and preferences. Certain medications can help to slow the progression of the disease, this is why caregivers must administer the right medication and dosage to avoid an unpleasant situation. Therapy and support groups may be beneficial to caregivers and family members to help alleviate stress and depression that comes with caring for someone with dementia.

Vascular Dementia: This is a very type of dementia but not as prevalent when compared to Alzheimer's disease. It is also known as post-stroke dementia and occurs when blood is restricted from flowing to the brain usually because of an arterial disease; thereby causes death in the brain cells. Vascular dementia is a broad term that describes problems with planning, judgment, reasoning, memory, and other thought processes caused by brain damage due to decreased blood flow to the brain. Memory loss and other symptoms of vascular dementia similar to Alzheimer's disease (AD) are easier to overcome with cues and reminders. Vascular dementia develops after a stroke blocks an artery in the brain, but strokes do not always cause vascular dementia, other conditions that damage blood vessels and reduce circulation, depriving the brain of oxygen and nutrients could be a contributing factor. These risk factors could increase vascular dementia: smoking, diabetes, heart disease, stroke, high cholesterol, or blood pressure. Vascular dementia symptoms vary depending on which part of the brain has poor blood flow. Caring for a patient with vascular dementia is not an easy task as the patient's case file must state the major risk factors to avoid a worse situation. Factors that increase the risk of heart disease and stroke, also increase the risk of vascular dementia. Controlling these risk factors may help reduce the likelihood of developing vascular dementia.

The health of the brain's blood vessels is linked to the health of the heart. A good heart and healthy brain is the best preventive measure to put vascular dementia under control. Another possible way to reduce your risk of dementia is to avoid the onset of type 2 diabetes through diet and exercise. Physical activity should be an important part of everyone's wellness plan. Maintaining normal blood pressure may aid in the prevention of dementia and other related diseases that comes with ageing. A series of strokes or ministrokes may be followed by a distinct pattern of vascular dementia symptoms. Unlike the gradual, steady decline seen in Alzheimer's disease dementia. Vascular disease and Alzheimer's disease frequently coexist. Strokes that block a brain artery usually result in a variety of symptoms, including vascular dementia. The risk of vascular dementia increases with the number of strokes that occur over time, both silent and apparent. High cholesterol levels have been linked to an increased risk of vascular dementia. Being overweight is a well-known risk factor for vascular diseases caregivers must ensure adequate nutrition to avoid diets with high cholesterol or poor food menu plans. High glucose levels harm the blood vessels this means that caregivers must consider the adverse effects of their patient's nutrition at all times.

The progression of vascular dementia is unpredictable, the symptoms could show up at any time. Vascular dementia appears to have different effects on different types of brain function, it impairs brain function such as reasoning, complex problem solving, or decision making it may take families longer to realize there is a problem. In Vascular dementia memory loss may not be a significant symptom depending on the severity of the blood vessel damaged or the location of the affected brain. These medical conditions must be avoided high cholesterol levels, lack of physical activity, diabetes, cardiovascular disease to reduce the risk of suffering from vascular dementia. People suffering from Type 2 diabetes are at a significantly higher risk of developing dementia. Women with diabetes have a 19% higher risk of developing vascular dementia than men. The genetic component of vascular dementia is not as well defined as it is in Alzheimer's disease. Cardiovascular risk factors, such as diabetes, have a genetic component that could increase the risk of vascular dementia. Controlling chronic health conditions lowers the risk of vascular dementia. As a caregiver, everything about your patient has to be under monitoring and evaluation to avoid the progression of vascular disease. To avoid the worsening of vascular dementia caregivers must adjust to changes in the patient's lifestyle and reduce the progression of dementia. Caregivers must ensure adequate rest, exercise and healthy diets for patients and themselves. Improving cardiovascular health physically, mental exercise with hearth healthy diets is beneficial to patients and caregivers. Vascular dementia can be managed to prevent further damage if diagnosed earlier, the sooner we intervene in someone's life, the more likely a positive outcome will occur. It must be done as soon as possible. It can't be after a string of strokes that could have been avoided. Alzheimer's drugs are less effective in treating vascular dementia. Family members should seek expert advice from a specialist when a person's heart or brain blood vessels are at risk. Stroke or heart attack is frequently the cause of death in patients with vascular dementia. Spending quality time and making sure a person with dementia is well-cared for and surrounded by people who love them could go a long way to alleviate the progression of the disease.

Dementia with Lewy bodies: This kind of Dementia is rare accounting for barely 10% of cases. It is usually caused by protein deposits in the cortex of the brain. Along with the symptoms of Alzheimer's disease, Lewy bodies can also cause hallucinations and insomnia. Lewy body dementia is the second most common type of progressive dementia, the disease is hard to diagnose. Lewy bodies are protein deposits that form in nerve cells in brain regions involved in the movement, thinking, and memory. About 1.4 million people in the United States suffer from Lewy Body Dementia, its symptoms can also be confused with other diseases and disorders. Lewy body dementia results in a progressive loss of mental abilities, visual hallucinations and changes in alertness and attention are common symptoms of Lewy body dementia. It's critical to be aware of Parkinson's-like symptoms such as tremors, rigid muscles, and slow movement as our loved one's or patients gets older. Lewy body dementia affects many parts of the brain, beginning with the grey matter or cerebral cortex, then the brain's outer layer. Changes in the nervous system caused by Lewy Body Dementia can lead to changes in behaviour and mood. If you or a loved one usually has a cheerful disposition or a mild temperament but has recently developed depression, anxiety, or paranoia, it may be time to see a doctor. Lewy body dementia affects the cerebral cortex responsible for perception, judgment, thought and communication by bringing impairments such as delusions, hallucinations, difficulty paying attention, and misidentification of objects. As the progression of this disease occurs more parts of the brain are affected and more symptoms such as difficulty forming new memories, difficulty moving and maintaining balance, difficulty sleeping or excessive sleepiness becomes visible.

Lewy body dementia comes in three stages: early, middle and late progressions. In the early stages of Lewy body dementia, the person may experience varied forms of restlessness, distortions, hallucinations, a REM sleep disorder where they act out their dreams and some movement difficulties. In the early progression of Lewy body dementia, some people may appear to freeze or become stuck while moving, while others may experience urinary urgency. In the middle stage progression of Lewy body dementia symptoms that resemble Parkinson's disease emerge, such as increased impairment of the body's motor functions. People suffering from the middle stage progression of the disease experience difficulty in speaking, falls, ability to swallow, increased delusions and paranoia thereby leading to decreased attention and prolonged periods of confusion. Lewy body dementia makes the patient very weak, caregiver's needs to watch out for pneumonia and other infections, which could affect a patient's quality of life. The late progression of Lewy body dementia results in extreme muscle rigidity and sensitivity to touch, at this stage almost all daily activities require some form of special care, speech is frequently difficult, whispered, or absent. Lewy Body Dementia hallucinations are typically vivid and visual, rather than auditory. Caregivers must be aware of cognitive fluctuations such as excessive weakness, struggle with focusing or concentrating on daily tasks. Please never force your patient suffering from dementia to stick to their routines, try to find out the cause for their forgetfulness or weakness.

Frontotemporal Dementia: This is a very rare kind of Dementia accounting for less than 5% of cases. Frontotemporal as the name implies, affects the frontal lobe of the brain responsible for planning, motivation and emotion. Frontotemporal dementia is a catch-all term for a group of rare brain disorders that primarily affects the brain regions commonly associated with personality, language, and behaviour. Depending on which part of the brain is affected some people with frontotemporal dementia experience dramatic personality changes, such as emotionally indifference, socially inappropriateness, or impulsive behaviours while others lose the ability to properly use language. Frontotemporal dementia is frequently misdiagnosed as a psychiatric disorder or Alzheimer's disease. Frontotemporal dementia typically manifests itself between the ages of 40 and 65, this is due to abnormal protein accumulation in the brain leading to deterioration and shrinkage of the frontal and temporal lobes. People suffering from Frontotemporal dementia experience difficulties in communication, Semantic dementia which impairs their ability to use and comprehend language, and struggle with planning and problem-solving abilities. They frequently appear to have grammar issues, such as leaving out or mixing up words, communicating with simpler, shorter, sometimes incomplete phrases. They gradually lose their ability to understand word meanings, recognize everyday objects, familiar faces, or use everyday items. Frontotemporal dementia can vary from person to person. The signs and symptoms worsen over time, usually over years. Caregivers need to watch out for compulsive repetitive behaviour, such as clapping, tapping, or smacking. Caring for a loved one with FTD can be extremely stressful for a caregiver. It is normal to feel denial, anger, and irritability. Caregivers may experience anxiety, depression, exhaustion, and other health issues. If caregivers notice any of these signs of stress, they should contact their healthcare provider. Please ensure as a caregiver you can help your patient with empathy and other interpersonal skills even if they do not understand what you are up to please remain calm with them.

Researchers have discovered that frontotemporal dementia and amyotrophic lateral sclerosis share genetics and molecular pathways (ALS). Frontotemporal dementia has been linked to several genetic mutations. However, more than half of those who develop frontotemporal dementia are vulnerable to infections and fall-related injuries. Dealing with Frontotemporal dementia can be frightening, frustrating, and embarrassing. Because some symptoms are uncontrollable, family members should not take their loved one's actions personally. Families must look after themselves while also ensuring that their loved one is treated with dignity and respect. People suffering from this disease may require round-the-clock nursing care or placement in an assisted living facility or nursing home. Caregivers should learn everything they can about frontotemporal dementia (FTD) and assemble a team of experts to assist the family in meeting the medical, financial, and emotional challenges they face. Healthcare providers, Home care nurses, social workers, neuropsychologists, speech and language therapists, financial advisors may be a part of the team that can assist in planning smooth future transitions for the patient and family members suffering from FTD or any form of dementia.

Mixed Dementia: Mixed Dementia is the occurrence of more than one type of dementia, usually Alzheimer's and vascular. It can also include other types. Mixed Dementia is a result of other health issues and stems from there. Mixed dementia is multifactorial, it is characterized by symptoms and abnormalities from more than one type of dementia at the same time. In most cases, mixed dementia is caused by a combination of Alzheimer's disease and vascular dementia or a combination of all dementia types known or unknown. Those suffering from mixed dementia may exhibit symptoms of Alzheimer's disease, vascular disease, and Lewy bodies. A clinical diagnosis of mixed dementia is difficult to obtain because scientists are unable to measure dementia-related brain changes in living individuals at this time. Although mixed dementia is diagnosed infrequently during life, many researchers believe it deserves more attention because the combination of two or more types of dementia-related brain changes may have a greater impact on the brain than just one type. Many researchers believe that a better understanding of mixed dementia, combined with the recognition that vascular changes are the most common coexisting brain change, could lead to a reduction in the number of people developing dementia. Controlling the overall risk factors for heart and blood vessel diseases may also protect the brain from vascular changes. Positive lifestyle changes, particularly during middle age, can play an important role in dementia prevention. Mentally stimulating activities such as memory exercises or learning a new language, eating healthy, maintaining a regular exercise routine, maintaining a socially active lifestyle, getting enough sleep, dealing with stress effectively, managing health issues such as high cholesterol, diabetes, and high blood pressure could go a long way in reducing the statistics for people suffering from dementia. Mixed dementia cannot be cured or slowed, risk reduction is one of the most important areas of dementia research at the moment.

CHAPTER 4

THE NASTY SIDE OF DEMENTIA.

Dementia usually occurs in stages and gets even worse even as more nerve cells are affected. However, it is best when the symptoms are discovered early so they can also be treated on time. Dementia symptoms vary depending on the cause, common signs and symptoms are cognitive shifts, personality changes, depressive disorder, psychological shifts, and anxiety. Consult a doctor if you or a loved one is experiencing memory problems or other dementia symptoms. Some treatable medical conditions can cause dementia symptoms, so it's critical to figure out what's causing them. One of the most difficult things to hear about dementia is that it is, in the majority of cases, irreversible and incurable. However, with early detection and treatment, the progression of some forms of dementia can be managed and slowed. Some doctors believe that an increase in the severity of the disease's signs and stages, such as mild, moderate, or severe dementia. However, because each individual is unique, all staging methods are based on symptoms; however, all systems describe early (and later) signs and symptoms can worsen over time. The cognitive decline that occurs with dementia conditions does not occur all at once; dementia progression varies in individuals. Dementia takes different forms and these forms have their individual triggers.

Dementia can be traced to three degenerative conditions namely: Neurological ailments, vascular conditions and diseases that affect the central nervous system. Neurological ailments include Huntington's disease, Corticobasal degeneration, and some kinds of multiple sclerosis, Parkinson's, and the most common cause - Alzheimer's disease. While vascular conditions generally conditions that affect the blood supply to the brain. Vascular dementia stems from this. Diseases that affect the central nervous system include Human immunodeficiency virus-related dementia, meningitis, Creutzfeldt-Jakob disease caused by infectious protein deposits in the brain. Risk factors for dementia stem across genes, age and gender. Age is the most common risk factor associated with Dementia. Statistics have shown that over 60% of young people develop Dementia at age 60 and above. This does not imply that Dementia is caused by ageing; it is only a high-risk factor. Alzheimer's disease as a form of dementia is prevalent in women more than men while vascular dementia is common in the male than female. There are several reasons for these variations. However, it is known that women tend to live longer than men. This essentially means that there are more elderly women than men. The genetics of Alzheimer's disease is quite complex. Findings have proven that 20 genes are associated with its occurrence.

One of the perks of taking care of a person with dementia is the high risk of verbal or physical assault. They might haul insults at you or even make false accusations about you. Some of them can even get physical especially if they feel threatened in any way.

It is important to understand that they do not mean or even know what they are saying. Dementia causes are deterioration in the brain, hence it is impossible for them to think straight. Never take what they say personally as they would do it to anyone else around them.

CHAPTER 5

SYMPTOMS OF CAREGIVER BURNOUT

Most people don't go into care with the intention of jeopardizing their own health. Those who care for a frail or needy loved one, on the other hand, are more likely to experience chronic stress and neglect self-care, both of which increase the risk of a variety of illnesses. As a result, the ability to continue providing high-quality care is harmed. Caregivers are known for having a unique personality: they are warm-hearted, sensitive, responsible, and well-intentioned. Burnout in caregivers is defined as mental, emotional, and physical tiredness caused by the responsibilities of supporting and caring for another person. Caregivers are frequently so preoccupied with the demands of the person they are caring for that they overlook their own health and well-being. Caregiver Burnout Signs and Symptoms are listed below.

A Fuse That Is Too Short: One clear symptom of caregiver stress is losing your temper or becoming enraged toward friends, family members, or even the person you're caring for. When significant or minor hurdles or challenges arise, frustration can rise dramatically.

Experiencing Emotional Outbursts: Another red flag is if you find yourself sobbing or feeling down more frequently than usual. Of course, it's natural to grieve if you're caring for a loved one who is deteriorating, and caregiving can bring up a variety of complex feelings. However, if you're becoming increasingly sensitive or feel emotionally vulnerable, there could be something more serious going on. Caregivers are at risk of depression. Emotional outbursts can be an unconscious release for emotions of overwhelm, even if you aren't clinically depressed.

Sleep Issues: Another indicator that you're having trouble getting asleep, staying asleep, or waking up tired is if you're having trouble falling asleep, staying asleep, or waking up exhausted. Caregiving, especially full-time caregiving, necessitates a lot of physical labour, but the emotions that come with it might keep you awake at night. On top of the exhausting labour you do all day, challenges your care recipient may be experiencing, such as straying or waking up in the middle of the night in discomfort, might cost you opportunities to relax. It can also be a vicious cycle, as tension, anxiety, and despair can make it difficult to fall or remain asleep.

Significant Weight Gain or Loss: Another indicator to look out for is sudden weight gain or loss. When people can't seem to find time to eat enough or nutritiously, stress might lead to weight loss. Anxiety suppresses appetite as well. Others acquire weight as a result of mindless or emotionally induced eating, frequent snacking, or quick but unhealthy meal choices as a result of feeling anxious or guilty.

Moody: Changes in food and sleeping patterns are other signs of sadness. If you've gained or lost more than five or 10 pounds since you started caring for others, your body may be signalling that you need help.

Physical Illnesses: Another red flag is if you're having more headaches or feeling like you're getting one cold after another. Alternatively, if you're experiencing chronic back or neck pain, or if you've got excessive blood pressure. Physical problems can be caused by mental and emotional stress. Stress, for example, might cause headaches that are more frequent, chronic, or severe than usual. You won't have the time or interest to adequately care for yourself, which will lead to increased stress. Stress reduces immunity, which may explain why caregivers have nearly twice the risk of chronic illnesses as non-caregivers.

Isolation from others: Burnout can also occur if you spend entire days with no one other than your care recipient or if you stop doing your regular activities to care for someone. If you're responsible for providing care, getting out can be difficult. You may believe you don't have enough time to pursue your previous interests. Changes in your care recipient's conduct may also make you feel ashamed or make going out in public too difficult. You may retreat, whether purposefully or unintentionally. Unfortunately, social isolation contributes to stress, although spending time with others and taking time for yourself is both restorative.

Family Dissatisfaction: It could be an indication of burnout if you're hearing more complaints from relatives or having more arguments with them. Taking up an entire load of care is a common caregiver temptation and mistake. It's also simple to convince ourselves that we have everything under control or that things aren't as bad as they appear. Denial is a strong feeling. It's difficult to recognize other options while you're in the middle of things. Even if you disagree, listening to an outsider might be beneficial. What may appear to be a critique or complaint may actually include a nugget of truth about your emotional well-being. While caregiving is difficult for everybody, some groups are more at risk of health problems and burnout than others, so it's vital to think about your specific challenges.

CHAPTER 6
ACTIVITIES TO EASE DEMENTIA.

Our memories can fail us as we become older, and our physical bodies can tire us out. For those with dementia, the issue is multiplied. People are frantically looking for things to do in order to lower their chances of developing dementia. Changing one's diet, tackling difficult brainteasers, exercising, meditating, and eating more veggies are all common strategies. More theories and strategies are being developed that may truly aid in the prevention of dementia in all of its forms. Seniors with Alzheimer's disease or another type of dementia, like everyone else, crave and benefit from connection and fulfilment. These exciting, interactive activities for dementia patients provide enjoyable, creative, and constructive ways to spend time with them. One strategy to delay the onset of dementia is to stay active and involved. Agitation, anxiety, despair, and rage are all reduced when you are pleasantly engaged in a gratifying task. It may potentially lessen the need for medicines by reducing problematic behaviours. Keeping dementia patients active in everyday activities and cognitively difficult occupations is good for both the body and the mind, and it can even halt the disease's progression in some situations. Staying active and involved might also help with dementia sleep issues. Dementia is a group of symptoms that gradually deteriorates a person's cognitive functioning, including crucial functions like remembering, thinking, and reasoning. Structured group activities are extremely rare to succeed. The most successful and useful sorts of activities for Alzheimer's are simple, brief activities offered several times a day. Housework and simple games can aid in the maintenance of motor skills. Music may also be a highly relaxing and entertaining activity. The individual, not the condition, should be the centre of attention. Make an effort to match them to activities that are appropriate for their background and expertise. Listed below are some activities that could help caretakers manage dementia symptoms.

Gardening: You can never go wrong with gardening, it is an exciting activity for people with dementia. It gives them the get outside (rather than staying indoors all day long) and the best opportunity to interact with other people. It brightens their mood and helps them breathe better. Gardening activities for the elderly, should not require much strain. Simple duties like weeding, watering can go a long way.

Bowling: Imagine the bowling ball as all of the stress and strain that has been building up in your life, and then release it violently to knock down the pins that represent the hurdles and challenges that you have faced. Bowling can be so much fun for people with dementia, especially when it involves other people.

Dancing: When we are happy sometimes we dance, jump and shout for joy. Dancing is a great way to alleviate stress and mood swings that dementia patients may experience. Dancing can also be done sitting and a good form of exercise to ease the joints.

Seated exercises: These exercises are ideal for ageing dementia patients as they require less stress. They can be carried out in one's home or in a group. Simple seated exercises include marching, clapping under the legs, raising of arms etc. These activities generally help to ease muscle movements.

Swimming: Swimming is a great sport for the elderly, it calms the nerves and makes one feel relaxed. Findings show that swimming can help reduce the occurrence of falls prevalent in dementia patients.

Walking: This is a great exercise for most people. Walking and exercise provide health benefits that go beyond the physical. Many people walk for mental and spiritual health as well as physical exercise. Take a vacation from your troubles inside. Observe your surroundings; appreciate the trees, flowers, birds, garden, or sky. Walks reduce boredom and engage the mind especially when carried out in groups.

Aerobics: Regular aerobic exercise will make a significant difference in your physique, metabolism, heart, and spirits. It has a one-of-a-kind ability to exhilarate and relax, to stimulate and soothe, to combat depression, and to relieve stress. Aerobics can be carried out at the early stages of dementia.

Small social events: Elder people usually face the risk of boredom. Little social events can keep them happy and full of life. It is important to ensure that these gatherings are not as large as dementia patients can be frightened by the crowd.

Puzzles and games: People in the early stage of dementia can still engage in activities that require them to use their brains. Statistics have also shown that continuous learning can reduce its risks. These activities include jigsaw puzzles, or even online puzzles, brain teasers and bingo. Bingo is an activity, designed for people specifically dealing with dementia. Caregivers can also engage in these activities with them to make it more fun.

Painting and drawing: This is a wonderful activity as it helps engage the mind and reduces stress. It can be done with family and caretakers. Keeping a visual diary is synonymous with withdrawing. You are free to draw whatever you like. Some people like to draw forms and things, while others like to draw animals or scenes. Art is utilized as a therapy medium as well as a means of expressing one's inner thoughts and feelings or their vision of the world around them.

Tai chi or qigong: These are types of Chinese martial arts that are calm and soothing. It is an activity that involves breathing and little body movement. This can help reduce strain and anxiety and improve sleep as well.

CHAPTER 7
CARING FOR DEMENTIA PATIENTS

Caregivers of a loved one with dementia suffer heightened health risks, according to studies. If you're caring for someone who has Alzheimer's disease or another dementia, your responsibility in handling daily duties will grow as the condition advances. Create a daily regimen. Some duties, such as showering or going to the doctor, are more manageable when the person is alert and refreshed. Allow aside some wiggle room for unexpected events or particularly trying days. Dementia does not take away a person's ability to interact with others, so use comedy to lighten the mood and potentially make them laugh and feel better. Caring for someone with dementia isn't always easy. It's counterintuitive. In fact, the logical thing isn't always the best option. Caring for someone can be physically and mentally exhausting because of the emotional toll it takes. Guilt, worry, and resentment are common feelings among long-term caregivers. All of these emotions are natural, but none of them is beneficial to your mental health. When you're taking care of someone else, it's easy to forget about yourself. Dementia causes people to become confused about reality and recall events that never happened. Avoid attempting to persuade them that they are incorrect. Be gentle, even if you know they're remembering something that didn't happen. Keep your attention on the emotions they're expressing and reply with comforting, supportive, and reassuring words and actions. Allow the person with dementia to do as much as they can with as little help as possible. For example, if you lay out clothes in the order they go on, he or she may be able to set the table with the use of visual cues or dress independently.

Limit exposures: Dementia patients can't handle so much information. This can get them tensed. When taking care of such patients, we should only engage them in light activities that do not require so many movements or thinking. If it TV shows, it shouldn't have many sounds or lights.

Keep communications simple as possible: It is very difficult for dementia patients to understand or communicate. Hence, when asked questions, we should make answers simple to understand and keep our questions to straight yes or no answers.

Set daily routines: Daily routines are quite easy to remember for dementia patients as it keeps them engaged and reduces stress and boredom. This helps reduce behavioural symptoms and reduces mood swings.

Dementia caregiver coping strategies: Every caregiver deserves a guide to coping with stress and burnout. The role of a caregiver generally involves administering care but this can be quite a herculean task with clients living with Dementia. As a result of the demands placed on the caregiver, he/she might experience burnouts that can impact one's emotional and physical health. In order to cope effectively, there are certain habits you can cultivate to reduce the stress and anxiety that comes with this care job.

CHAPTER 8

THERAPY FOR DEMENTIA CAREGIVERS

It's typical for people to be resistant to the concept of seeking counselling or other mental health care, regardless of their function in life. Sometimes this resistance creates a strong enough barrier that people are unable to receive the assistance that would make a significant difference in their life and the lives of those around them. Stress and burnout among dementia caregivers can be a major reason for seeking help from a therapist, as well as a major reason for avoiding seeking help. Seeking help and then receiving it may appear to be simply another item on an already long list of obligations. Furthermore, caregiver stress might be challenging enough, and you may be hesitant to dig out more of the issues that counselling would encourage. However, one common symptom of caregiver burnout is that stress builds up and is pushed down, allowing more to build up. Avoiding it does not make it go away; it only adds to the tension and agony. Depression in dementia carers is a very real and dangerous disorder that could greatly benefit from ongoing treatment. Even if it is judged necessary, finding the time and separation from your ageing loved one to seek this kind of assistance can be tough. However, there are always resources and services available to help dementia caregiver's deal with unique issues and reduce stress. In fact, you may be able to have a skilled therapist come to you.

Meditation Course with a Guide: Burnout can strike any caregiver at any time. Even the most seasoned caretakers can overwork themselves and become sad, worried, and unmotivated as a result. You must set aside time for yourself in order to avoid burnout. Meditation is one of the most effective strategies to alleviate the stress that comes with dementia caregiving. Downloading an app, purchasing a CD/DVD, or renting one from the library are all options for guided meditation courses. Take a few minutes each day to deepen your breathing, ease worry, and practice self-care.

Make a request for assistance: You can't do it all by yourself. To help with the daily load of caregiving, reach out to other family members, friends, or volunteer organizations. Schedule numerous pauses throughout the day to pursue your hobbies and interests while also keeping track of your personal health requirements. This is not being unfaithful or neglectful to your partner. Caregivers who take regular breaks not only provide greater care, but they also enjoy their roles as caregivers more. A caregiver's support network may be the most crucial tool in their armoury. You should have a support system of friends and family members who can assist you with caregiving responsibilities like running errands, remaining with your senior loved one while you go to yoga class, or listening to you complain about your day. Don't be hesitant to ask for help from your friends and family; you might be surprised at how willing they are to help.

Changing Your Mindset: Try rethinking your issue in ways that lessen frustration as you take some time to collect your thoughts. How you think has a big impact on how you feel. Frustration is, of course, a natural reaction to challenging circumstances. If you examine your reaction to a frustrating circumstance, you will almost always discover some type of maladaptive or negative thinking that serves to increase your irritation while also keeping you from objectively assessing the problem and finding a better method to deal with it.

Become a member of a support group: You'll be able to learn from the mistakes and successes of others who have experienced similar difficulties. Connecting with individuals who understand what you're going through might also make you feel less alone, afraid, and hopeless.

Maintain a social life: Make time for your friends so that they don't vanish. You may be feeling isolated or irritated because your old circle no longer seems to care about you and how you're doing. But is it possible that you've turned them down so many times because of your caregiving responsibilities, or that they've gotten the impression that you're just not interested in them because you've turned them down so many times because of your caregiving responsibilities? So, when you do see them, don't just talk about caring for them. If every conversation is about the same topic, it's a sign that that topic is taking over your life.

Go on vacation: Vacations are difficult to plan when you have a disabled or impaired person to consider, but being unable to recall the last time you took a break is a sure sign you're overdue. It is not necessary to spend three weeks in France. If you must start small: a simple overnight at a friend's house or a nearby resort. Simply do something. Caregiving stress can be reduced by taking breaks from caregiving.

Develop a hobby: Your hobby does not have to be traditional, such as stamp collecting or bird watching; it simply needs to be a distraction from caregiving. Reading trashy novels, taking up knitting, joining a book club, taking adult education courses, being a matinée-movie addict, or simply spending time with your children and grandchildren all count. Anything that takes you away from caregiving for bursts of time. Bonus points if it also gets you out of the house.

Learn to set emotional and practical limits in your caregiver relationship: A therapist can help you recognize that, while it's critical to give yourself space to experience the emotions that arise, they're just that: emotions. When we strive to ignore or avoid particular feelings entirely, we often find that those sentiments become even stronger. We may even begin to identify with or be controlled by such feelings.

Apps for Health: Apps are a lifesaver for today's carer. Keep track of your patient's or loved one's prescriptions with an app like Medisafe if they have many drugs to take every day. Download an app like Instant Heart Rate if you need to take your loved one's vitals on a regular basis. If you want to keep track of your health as well, there are apps that can assist you to do so.

CONCLUSION

Dementia can be managed. Making health-care decisions for someone who is no longer capable of doing so can be difficult. That is why it is critical to plan ahead of time for health care directives. Learning about your loved one's disease will help you understand what to expect and what you can do as the dementia progresses.

Seek Help: When you require assistance, ask for it. This could include enlisting the assistance of family and friends, as well as contacting local services for additional care requirements.

Stay healthy: Consume nutritious foods to help you stay healthy and active for a longer period of time.

Be active: Participate in an online or in-person caregiver support group. Meeting other caregivers allows you to share stories and ideas, which can help you feel less isolated.

Communication: It is difficult for people with Alzheimer's and related dementias because they have trouble remembering things. Reassure the person. Speak clearly and calmly. Pay attention to his or her worries and frustrations. If the person is angry or afraid, try to demonstrate that you understand.

Be Awesome: Be the best caregiver at all times. Please ensure you conduct yourself properly with patience and good work ethics.

www.ingramcontent.com/pod-product-compliance
Lightning Source LLC
Chambersburg PA
CBHW070335240526
45466CB00027B/1992